Strong Core, Radiant You: The Ultimate Guide to Female Abs Workouts and how to sculpt and Strengthen Your Core.

By

Melissa A. Pinkston

Copyright Page:

© 2023 [Melissa A. Pinkston]

All rights reserved. No part of this publication may be reproduced, distributed, or transmitted in any form or by any means, including photocopying, recording, or other electronic or mechanical methods, without the prior written permission of the publisher, except in the case of brief quotations embodied in critical reviews and certain other noncommercial uses permitted by copyright law. For permission requests, write to the publisher at the address below.

Disclaimer:

The information provided in this book is for general informational purposes only and is not intended as medical advice. Before beginning any fitness program, including the exercises and suggestions presented in this book, it is advisable to consult with a qualified healthcare professional. The author and publisher disclaim any responsibility for any adverse effects or consequences resulting from the use or application of the information contained in this book.

Every effort has been made to ensure that the information in this book is accurate and up-to-date. However, the author and publisher do not warrant or represent that the information is free from errors or omissions. The author and publisher accept no responsibility or liability for any injuries, losses, or damages arising from the use of the exercises, advice, or information presented in this book.

Names, characters, businesses, places, events, and incidents are either the products of the author's imagination or used in a fictitious manner. Any resemblance to actual persons, living or dead, or actual events is purely coincidental.

About the Author:

In the pulsating heartbeat of the fitness world, where determination meets passion, you'll find Melissa A. Pinkston, the vibrant architect behind "Strong Core, Radiant You." But let's rewind to where this inspiring journey began.

Born into a whirlwind of energy, Melissa A. Pinkston wasn't always the epitome of fitness. In fact, her tryst with the gym began as a reluctant dance. Picture a young woman navigating the labyrinth of conflicting fitness advice, tirelessly trying to sculpt her own path to wellness. This was the genesis of an extraordinary transformation that would ultimately shape the essence of this book.

In the bustling city where skyscrapers touch the clouds, Melissa A. Pinkston found her sanctuary in the gym. However, her evolution was far from a linear ascent. Imagine a protagonist in a novel, facing setbacks, moments of self-doubt, and the challenge of navigating uncharted territories. This was Melissa A. Pinkston's narrative.

Her journey mirrored the struggles many women face – the quest for a strong core, not just for aesthetics but as a symbol of resilience. It was during the sweat-soaked hours, amidst the clinks of weights and echoes of motivational beats, that Melissa A. Pinkston discovered the transformative power of core workouts.

As her muscles grew stronger, so did her spirit. The gym became a metaphorical cocoon where Melissa A. Pinkston underwent a metamorphosis. The desire to share this empowering experience with fellow women, to guide them through the labyrinth she had conquered, ignited the spark to pen down "Strong Core, Radiant You."

This book is not just a collection of exercises; it's an anthology of Melissa A. Pinkston's unwavering determination, sprinkled with the magic of her unique journey. Each page carries the echoes of her personal triumphs and the echoes of the countless women she has inspired along the way.

Beyond the pages, Melissa A. Pinkston is not just an author but a mentor, a beacon of strength, and an advocate for every woman seeking to redefine her boundaries. So, as you embark on this transformative journey through "Strong Core, Radiant You," remember that the woman behind the words is more than an author – she's a storyteller of resilience, an architect of strength, and your companion on the path to a more radiant you.

Table of Content

Introduction

Welcome to "Strong Core, Radiant You: The Ultimate Guide to Female Abs Workouts." In the journey towards optimal health and fitness, a strong core stands as the foundation of your strength and vitality. This book is not just about sculpting abs; it's a holistic approach to empowering women through targeted exercises, valuable insights, and a commitment to well-being.

As we delve into the world of core workouts, we'll uncover the anatomy of the core muscles, explore the myriad benefits they offer, and equip you with a comprehensive toolkit of exercises. Whether you're a beginner taking the first steps on your fitness journey or someone seeking advanced challenges, this guide is crafted to meet you where you are.

Prepare to embrace a transformative experience, where each chapter unfolds a new dimension of core strength. Beyond the physical aspects, we'll discuss the significance of consistency, proper nutrition, and the mental resilience that accompanies a strong core.

Join me in this empowering journey as we sculpt and strengthen not just your core but the radiant, resilient you. It's time to embark on a path that goes beyond aesthetics — a path that leads to a healthier, more confident, and empowered version of yourself. Let's get started on building a strong core for a vibrant and radiant you!

In the realm of women's health and fitness, the core isn't just a set of muscles; it's the powerhouse of vitality, the epicenter of strength that radiates throughout your entire being. Understanding the profound significance of a strong core is like unlocking the secret to a more vibrant and empowered life.

Your core, encompassing muscles from the abdomen to the lower back and hips, is not merely a visual centerpiece. It's your body's stabilizing force, the linchpin supporting every movement, whether you're conquering a challenging workout, gracefully navigating your day, or embracing life's unexpected twists and turns.

Why is a Strong Core Vital for Women?

1. Posture and Elegance:

A strong core is the anchor for graceful posture. Picture yourself standing tall with confidence, shoulders back, and an air of elegance – that's the gift of a robust core. It's not just about standing straight; it's about embodying your strength with poise.

2. Balance and Stability:

As life throws its curveballs, both figuratively and literally, your core is your stability compass. From conquering yoga poses to navigating uneven terrains, a strong core provides the stability needed for balance in every aspect of your life.

3. Functional Fitness:

Ever find yourself lifting groceries, reaching for something on a high shelf, or playing with your kids? Your core is at the center of these everyday movements. A strengthened core ensures that your body functions optimally, making these activities not only effortless but enjoyable.

4. Pain Prevention and Spinal Health:

A well-conditioned core acts as a protective shield for your spine. It helps prevent back pain and supports your spine's natural curvature, allowing you to move with freedom and reduce the risk of injuries.

5. Empowerment and Confidence:

Beyond the physical, a strong core fosters a sense of internal empowerment. It's not just about looking good; it's about feeling strong from within. Imagine the confidence that radiates when you know your core is a resilient force that can weather any storm.

As we embark on this journey through "Strong Core, Radiant You," remember that it's not just about sculpting abs; it's about cultivating a foundation of strength that transcends the physical. Your core is your ally in the pursuit of holistic health and fitness, and this book is your guide to unlocking its transformative power. Let's delve deeper into the world of female abs workouts and discover the radiant you that awaits beneath the surface.

Core Anatomy

Step into the heart of empowerment, where the essence of "Strong Core, Radiant You" takes on a deeper resonance. Core Anatomy is not just a lesson in anatomy; it's a journey of self-discovery, a warm embrace of the incredible symphony playing within you.

Embarking on an Inner Voyage:

Picture your core as a canvas, painted with muscles that tell a story of resilience, strength, and potential. As we venture into the intricate landscapes of your core anatomy, let this be a moment of revelation—a celebration of the remarkable ensemble residing within.

A Symphony of Movement and Stability:

Think of your core as a living symphony, each muscle playing its unique melody, harmonizing movement and stability. In understanding this symphony, you're not just learning; you're composing a masterpiece of strength that resonates in every step, every stretch, and every breath.

Beyond the Six-Pack Fantasy:

Uncover the magic beyond aesthetics. As we navigate the realms of core anatomy, you're not just sculpting muscles; you're sculpting a deeper connection with your body. This chapter is an invitation to embrace your inner orchestra, to dance with the rhythm of your own strength.

So, as we journey into the intricacies of your core's anatomy, may you feel the warmth of self-discovery, the thrill of understanding, and the empowering embrace of a body that tells a story of strength. Join me in Chapter 2 as we embark on an inner voyage, exploring the wonders of your core—the beating heart of your radiant self.

Meet Your Muscular Maestros:

1. Rectus Abdominis:
Your Frontline Warriors: Beyond the pursuit of sculpted abs, these muscles are storytellers of forward flexion and abdominal compression. They embody the beauty of strength in simplicity.
Location:Front and center, this is the muscle responsible for the coveted six-pack appearance.
Function:Responsible for flexing the spine and compressing the abdomen. Often referred to as the "six-pack" muscles, they play a role in forward movement.

2. Obliques (Internal and External):
Dancers of the Side:Let's waltz with the obliques, masters of rotation and lateral flexion. They bring a dynamic elegance to your core, infusing it with grace and versatility.
Location: Along the sides of your torso
Function: Facilitate rotation, lateral flexion, and stabilization. Internal obliques aid in torso rotation, while external obliques assist in side bending and rotation.

3. Transverse Abdominis:
The Core's Corset: Deep within, this muscle embraces your organs like a protective corset. It's the silent powerhouse, offering stability and support to your entire core.
Function: Acts like a natural weight belt, providing stability and support to the spine and pelvis. It plays a crucial role in maintaining abdominal tension and supporting internal organs.

4. Erector Spinae:

Backstage Champions:Often in the shadows, these muscles contribute to spinal extension and posture. They are the unsung heroes, ensuring your back stands tall with resilience.

Location: Along the spine

Function:Located along the spine, these muscles are responsible for spinal extension, helping you stand upright. They contribute to maintaining proper posture and supporting the back during movement.

5. Pelvic Floor Muscles:

Foundation of Grace: Below the pelvis, these muscles provide the foundational support for your pelvic organs, ensuring not just strength but a graceful balance from within.

Function:Located below the pelvis, these muscles support pelvic organs, contribute to bladder control, and play a vital role in stabilizing the core.

Understanding the functions of these key core muscles is essential for tailoring effective workouts and promoting overall core strength and stability. Each muscle contributes to the intricate balance that forms the foundation of a strong and resilient core.

Unlocking the Power Within:
The Transformative Benefits of a Strong Core for Women

In the tapestry of our lives, our core stands as a silent hero, weaving together the threads of strength, resilience, and vitality. As we embark on the exploration of the profound benefits that a strong core bestows upon women, envision it not merely as a pursuit of aesthetics but as a journey towards holistic well-being, a journey that transcends the boundaries of the gym and echoes through the rhythms of everyday life.

Posture: The Silent Symphony of Strength

Posture is not just about standing tall; it's a reflection of the inner strength that radiates from your core. A strong core acts as a sculptor, shaping the canvas of your body into a masterpiece of grace and poise. Picture this: navigating a crowded room with confidence, shoulders back, and a spine that effortlessly supports your stature. A strong core isn't just about aesthetics; it's your ally in projecting an image of confidence and self-assurance.

Consider the professional woman, juggling responsibilities, moving through the corporate landscape with grace. Her strong core is the anchor that ensures she stands tall, not just physically, but also metaphorically, in the face of challenges. It's the unspoken language of authority, the posture that says, "I am here, I am capable, and I am unyielding."

Balance: The Dance of Stability

Life is a constant dance, and balance is the choreography that keeps us moving forward. A strong core is the dance partner that ensures your every step is taken with poise and stability. Picture yourself gracefully moving through a yoga sequence, effortlessly transitioning from one pose to another. It's not just about flexibility; it's about the core's role in maintaining equilibrium.

In the world of a busy mom, balance isn't just a physical act but a metaphor for managing the delicate dance of daily life. From carrying groceries with ease to chasing after a playful child, a strong core ensures stability in motion. It's the unspoken assurance that every step is grounded, every movement purposeful, and every balance maintained with grace.

Daily Activities: From Mundane to Extraordinary

Our daily activities, seemingly mundane, become extraordinary feats when viewed through the lens of a strong core. Imagine the simple act of bending down to tie your shoelaces. It's not just a task; it's a showcase of the core's ability to provide support and flexibility, making even the smallest actions a testament to your physical prowess.

Now, envision the adventurous spirit exploring the outdoors – hiking through rugged terrains, reveling in the freedom of movement. A strong core is the compass guiding each step, ensuring not just the thrill of the journey but the resilience to face the challenges it presents.

From lifting a suitcase into an overhead compartment to the nuanced dance of mastering a new dance routine, every activity becomes an opportunity for your core to shine. It's not about isolating the strength of your midsection; it's about integrating it into the symphony of your life, where every note is a testament to your core's unwavering support.

 A Radiant You Beyond Repose

As we conclude this exploration into the manifold benefits of a strong core for women, envision a future where strength is not just a pursuit but a lifestyle. A lifestyle where your posture exudes confidence, your balance navigates the complexities of life, and your daily activities become a showcase of resilience.

Let this journey into the realm of core strength be an invitation – an invitation to embrace the transformative power within. As you navigate the intricate dance of life, may your strong core be the unwavering partner, guiding you with grace, stability, and a radiant strength that transcends the boundaries of the physical into the tapestry of your everyday existence. Here's to a journey where the benefits of a strong core become the melody of your life, echoing with vitality and radiance in every step you take.

Getting Started:
Your Journey to Core Strength

Congratulations on taking the first step towards a stronger, more vibrant you! This is your gateway to the world of core workouts—a realm where determination meets guidance. Whether you're a newcomer to fitness or returning after a hiatus, this chapter is tailored to set the foundation for a transformative journey. Let's dive into the essentials of getting started, emphasizing the importance of proper form and the crucial role of warm-up exercises.

Embarking on the Journey: Tips for Beginners

1. Start Slow, Progress Steadily:

As you begin your core workout journey, resist the urge to dive into advanced exercises. Begin with fundamental movements to allow your body to adapt gradually. Progression is the key – it's not about where you start, but how far you can go.

2. Listen to Your Body:

Pay attention to your body's signals. If you experience discomfort beyond the typical muscle engagement, pause and reassess. It's crucial to differentiate between the burn of a good workout and the strain of improper form.

3. Focus on Form Over Intensity:

Quality trumps quantity. Ensure your movements are precise, engaging the targeted muscles. Proper form not only maximizes effectiveness but also minimizes the risk of injury. Consider it the blueprint for sculpting a strong and resilient core.

4. Breathe Mindfully:

Incorporate conscious breathing into your workouts. Oxygen fuels your muscles and helps maintain focus. Inhale during the easier phase of the exercise and exhale during the effort, creating a rhythm that enhances both performance and mindfulness.

5. Variety is Key:

Keep your routine dynamic by incorporating a variety of exercises. This not only prevents monotony but also ensures a comprehensive approach to core development. From planks to leg raises, diversity is the spice that ignites progress.

The Importance of Proper Warm-Up: Preparing Your Core for Action

1. Increased Blood Flow:

A proper warm-up boosts blood circulation to the muscles, preparing them for the demands of your workout. This increased blood flow enhances flexibility and reduces the risk of injury.

2. Joint Mobilization:

Warm-up exercises gently mobilize your joints, enhancing their range of motion. This is particularly crucial for core workouts, where flexibility contributes to effective engagement of abdominal muscles.

3. Activation of Core Muscles:

Include exercises that activate the core during warm-up. This primes the muscles for the workload ahead, creating a mind-body connection that sets the stage for optimal performance.

4. Mental Preparation:

Warm-up is not only physical but also mental preparation. It provides a few moments to shift your focus from the outside world to the present workout, fostering a mindful approach to each movement.

Crafting Your Warm-Up Routine:

Cardio Burst: 5–10 minutes of light cardio, such as brisk walking or jumping jacks, to elevate your heart rate.

Jumping jack

Here's a step-by-step guide on how to perform jumping jacks with proper form:

1. Starting Position:
   - Stand upright with your feet together and arms resting at your sides. This is your initial position.

2. Jumping Phase:
   - Simultaneously jump and spread your legs apart while raising your arms overhead. Your arms should form a "V" shape.
   - Keep your knees slightly bent to absorb the impact as you land.

3. Landing Phase:
   - Quickly reverse the motion by jumping back to the starting position.
   - Bring your feet together and lower your arms back to your sides.

4. *Repeat:
   - Continue the motion in a rhythmic and continuous manner.

Tips for Proper Form:

1. Maintain Core Engagement:
   - Keep your core muscles tight throughout the exercise. This not only enhances the effectiveness of the movement but also supports your lower back.

2. Land Softly:
   - Land on the balls of your feet to minimize impact on your joints. Absorb the landing by slightly bending your knees.

3. Controlled Movements:
   - Execute the exercise with controlled movements. Avoid flinging your arms or legs excessively, ensuring a smooth and controlled motion.

4. Breathing:
   - Coordinate your breath with the movement. Inhale as you spread your arms and legs, and exhale as you return to the starting position.

Dynamic Stretching: Engage in dynamic stretches that target your core, such as torso twists and leg swings

Leg swings
Leg Swings: A Dynamic Prelude to Limber Limbs

Let's dive into the step-by-step guide to master this graceful and beneficial movement:

1. Initial Position:

   - Begin by standing tall with your feet hip-width apart. Engage your core for stability.

2. Front-to-Back Swings:

   - Holding onto a sturdy support (such as a wall or a bar), shift your weight to one leg.

   - Swing the opposite leg forward and backward in a controlled motion. Keep the movement within a comfortable range, avoiding overextension.

3. Side-to-Side Swings:

   - Still holding onto the support, swing the leg out to the side and back toward the center. Ensure controlled movement to maintain balance.

4. Lateral Swings:

   - With the support on your side, swing your leg across your body and back to the starting position. This targets the inner and outer thighs.

5. Repeat on the Other Leg:

   - Once you've completed the swings on one leg, switch to the other. Perform a balanced number of swings on each leg.

Tips for Proper Form:

1. Controlled Movements:

   - Execute each swing with control, avoiding abrupt or jerky movements. This ensures you're actively engaging the muscles throughout the range of motion.

2. Maintain Posture:

- Keep your upper body upright, shoulders relaxed, and core engaged. This promotes stability and prevents unnecessary strain on your lower back.

3. Gradual Increase in Intensity:

- Begin with smaller swings and gradually increase the range of motion as your muscles warm up. Listen to your body and adapt the intensity accordingly.

4. Flex the Toes:

- Point your toes forward during the front-to-back swings and flex them during the lateral swings. This engages different muscle groups, enhancing the stretch.

Activation Exercises:Perform light core activation exercises, like gentle planks or pelvic tilts.

Your Journey Begins Here

Armed with these tips for beginners, remember that every journey begins with a single step. Your commitment, coupled with mindful practices, will be the compass guiding you through this transformative expedition. As you lace up your metaphorical workout shoes, let the essence of this chapter be the wind beneath your wings, propelling you towards a stronger, more radiant version of yourself. The journey to core strength is a personal odyssey, and with each step, you're crafting a narrative of empowerment and resilience. Let the adventure unfold!

The Power of Planks:
Sculpting Your Core Foundation

Welcome to the chapter that's about to revolutionize your core workout – Chapter 5, dedicated to the almighty plank. Brace yourself for an exploration into the diverse world of plank exercises, each one a secret weapon in your arsenal for sculpting a resilient and toned core. Let's dive deep into the realm of planks, understanding their instructions, variations, and the specific parts of your core that they skillfully target.

1. Standard Plank:

Starting Position: Begin in a push-up position, arms straight and directly beneath your shoulders.
Execution: Engage your core, forming a straight line from head to heels. Hold for the desired duration, ensuring your body remains rigid.
Core Focus: Rectus abdominis, transverse abdominis, obliques, erector spinae.
Duration:
    Beginner: 20-30 seconds
    Intermediate: 30-60 seconds
    Advanced: 60 seconds or more

2. Side Plank:

Starting Position: Lie on your side, supporting your upper body on your elbow and forearm.
Execution: Lift your hips until your body forms a straight line from head to heels. Hold the position on each side.
 Core Focus: Obliques, transverse abdominis, erector spinae.
Duration(per side):
   Beginner: 15-20 seconds
   Intermediate: 20-40 seconds
   Advanced: 40 seconds or more

3. Reverse Plank:

Starting Position: Sit on the floor with your legs extended in front of you, hands placed behind you.
Execution: Lift your hips, creating a straight line from head to heels. Hold the position, engaging your core and keeping your body aligned.
Core Focus: Rectus abdominis, transverse abdominis, hip flexors.
Duration:
   Beginner: 15-30 seconds
   Intermediate: 30-45 seconds
   Advanced: 45 seconds or more

4. Plank with Shoulder Taps:

Starting Position: Assume a standard plank position.

Execution: While maintaining the plank, tap your left shoulder with your right hand and vice versa. Alternate taps.
Core Focus: Obliques, transverse abdominis.
Duration:
   Beginner: 20-30 seconds
   Intermediate: 30-45 seconds
   Advanced: 45 seconds or more

5. Plank to Downward Dog:

Starting Position: Begin in a plank position.
Execution: Lift your hips towards the ceiling, forming an inverted V shape. Return to the plank position and repeat.
Core Focus: Rectus abdominis, shoulders, hamstrings.
Duration:
   Beginner: 20-30 seconds
   Intermediate: 30-45 seconds
   Advanced: 45 seconds or more

6. Spiderman Plank:

Starting Position: In a plank position, bring your right knee towards your right elbow.
Execution: Return to the plank position and repeat on the other side.
Core Focus: Obliques, transverse abdominis, hip flexors.
Duration:
   Beginner: 15-20 seconds
   Intermediate: 20-40 seconds
   Advanced: 40 seconds or more

7. High Plank to Low Plank:

Starting Position: Begin in a high plank.
Execution: Lower your body into a forearm plank one arm at a time, then return to the starting position.
Core Focus: Entire core, including the rectus abdominis, transverse abdominis, and obliques.
Duration:
  Beginner: 20-30 seconds
  Intermediate: 30-45 seconds
  Advanced: 45 seconds or more

Variations are the Spice of Progress:
Feel free to modify these plank exercises based on your fitness level. If you're a beginner, start with shorter durations and gradually increase. For the seasoned plank enthusiasts, challenge yourself with longer holds or incorporate these variations into a high-intensity circuit. Remember, it's essential to prioritize proper form over duration. As you progress, you can gradually increase the duration to continue challenging your core muscles. Listen to your body, and feel free to adjust the durations based on your individual fitness level and goals.

Abdominal Crunches Mastery: *A Symphony of Core Strength*

Welcome to the chapter that unveils the art and science of abdominal crunches. Chapter 6 is your guide to mastering the intricacies of crunch variations, understanding their targeted benefits, and sculpting a core that radiates strength. Let's embark on a journey through different crunch variations, explore the specific parts of the core they engage, delve into suggested durations, and learn the precise execution of each exercise.

1. Standard Abdominal Crunch:

  Core Focus: Primarily targets the rectus abdominis.
  Duration:
   Beginner:20-30 crunches
   Intermediate: 30-50 crunches
   Advanced: 50 crunches or more

Execution:

- Lie on your back with your knees bent and feet flat on the floor.

- Place your hands gently behind your head, avoiding any pulling on your neck.

- Engage your core, lift your shoulders off the floor, and exhale as you crunch towards your knees.

- Inhale as you lower your upper back to the starting position.

2. Bicycle Crunch:

Core Focus: Engages the rectus abdominis, obliques, and hip flexors.

Duration:

Beginner: 15-20 repetitions (each side)

Intermediate: 20-30 repetitions (each side)

Advanced: 30 repetitions (each side) or more

Execution:

- Start in a standard crunch position.

- Bring your right knee towards your chest while simultaneously twisting your torso to bring your left elbow towards your right knee.

- Straighten your right leg as you bring your left knee towards your chest, twisting to bring your right elbow towards your left knee.

- Continue in a pedaling motion.

3. Reverse Crunch:

Core Focus: Targets the lower abdominal muscles.
Duration:
  Beginner: 15-20 crunches
  Intermediate: 20-30 crunches
  Advanced: 30 crunches or more

Execution:
  - Lie on your back with your hands at your sides or under your hips for support.
  - Lift your legs towards the ceiling, keeping them straight.
  - Engage your lower abs to lift your hips off the floor, bringing your legs towards your face.
  - Lower your legs back down without letting them touch the floor.

4. Russian Twist:

  Core Focus: Emphasizes the obliques and transverse abdominis.
  Duration:
  Beginner: 15-20 twists (each side)
  Intermediate: 20-30 twists (each side)
  Advanced: 30 twists (each side) or more

Execution:
  - Sit on the floor with your knees bent and feet flat.
  - Lean back slightly, keeping your back straight, and engage your core.
  - Twist your torso to the right, then to the left, tapping the floor beside you with each twist.

5. Vertical Leg Crunch:

Core Focus: Targets the rectus abdominis and improves upper abdominal definition.
Duration:
Beginner: 15-20 crunches
Intermediate: 20-30 crunches
Advanced: 30 crunches or more

Execution:
- Lie on your back with your legs extended towards the ceiling.
- Crunch your upper body towards your legs, lifting your shoulders off the floor.
- Lower your upper body back down without letting it rest completely.

6. Oblique Crunch:

Core Focus: Isolates the obliques, enhancing waistline definition.
Duration:
Beginner: 15-20 crunches (each side)
Intermediate: 20-30 crunches (each side)
Advanced: 30 crunches (each side) or more

Execution:
- Lie on your back with your knees bent and feet flat.
- Place your hands behind your head and twist your torso, bringing your right elbow towards your left knee.

- Repeat on the other side.

7. Pilates Scissor:

Core Focus: Engages the entire core, especially targeting the lower abs.
Duration:
Beginner: 15-20 repetitions (each leg)
Intermediate: 20-30 repetitions (each leg)
Advanced: 30 repetitions (each leg) or more

Execution:
- Lie on your back with your legs extended towards the ceiling.
- Lower one leg towards the floor while keeping the other leg lifted.
- Switch legs in a scissor-like motion, engaging your lower abs throughout.

Tips for Precise Execution:

1. Mindful Control:
- Focus on controlled movements, ensuring that your core muscles do the work rather than relying on momentum.

2. Neck and Head Position:
- Keep your neck and head in a neutral position to avoid strain. Imagine holding an apple between your chin and chest.

3. Breathe Mindfully:

   - Exhale during the upward phase of the crunch and inhale during the downward phase to maintain a rhythmic breathing pattern.

4. Engage the Core:

   - Throughout each exercise, consciously engage your core muscles. This ensures optimal activation and effectiveness.

Now that you have the keys to executing each crunch variation with precision, let the symphony of abdominal crunches sculpt your core into a masterpiece of strength and definition. Adjust the suggested durations based on your fitness level, and always prioritize proper form for optimal results. Happy crunching!

Leg Raises and Lower Ab Workouts:
Elevating Core Strength

Prepare to embark on a journey dedicated to sculpting the often elusive lower abdominal muscles. Chapter 7 is your guide to leg raises and targeted lower ab workouts, a key component in achieving a well-rounded and defined core. Let's delve into exercises specifically designed to target the lower abs, uncover their targeted benefits, explore suggested durations, and master the precise execution of each exercise.

1. Leg Raises:

Core Focus: Targets the lower abs, engaging the rectus abdominis.
Duration:
Beginner: 15-20 repetitions

Intermediate: 20-30 repetitions
Advanced: 30 repetitions or more

Execution:
- Lie on your back with your legs extended.
- Keep your hands at your sides or under your hips for support.
- Lift your legs towards the ceiling, maintaining straight and controlled movements.
- Lower your legs back down without letting them touch the floor.

2. Reverse Crunch with Hip Raise:

Core Focus: Engages the lower abs and hip flexors.
Duration:
Beginner: 15-20 repetitions
Intermediate: 20-30 repetitions
Advanced: 30 repetitions or more

Execution:
- Lie on your back with your hands at your sides.
- Lift your legs towards the ceiling, then curl your hips off the floor.
- Lower your hips back down without letting your legs touch the floor.

3. Scissor Kicks:

Core Focus: Targets the lower abs and hip flexors.
Duration:

Beginner: 20-30 seconds
Intermediate: 30-45 seconds
Advanced: 45 seconds or more

Execution:
- Lie on your back with your hands under your hips.
- Lift your legs slightly off the ground.
- Perform a scissor-like motion, crisscrossing your legs in controlled movements.

4. Mountain Climbers:

Core Focus: Engages the lower abs, hip flexors, and obliques.
Duration:
Beginner: 20-30 seconds
Intermediate: 30-45 seconds
Advanced: 45 seconds or more

Execution:
- Start in a plank position with your hands directly under your shoulders.
- Bring one knee towards your chest, then switch legs in a dynamic, alternating fashion.

5. Hanging Leg Raises:

Core Focus: Targets the lower abs and challenges overall core stability.
Duration:
Beginner: 10-15 repetitions

Intermediate: 15-20 repetitions
Advanced: 20 repetitions or more

Execution:
- Hang from a pull-up bar with your arms fully extended.
- Lift your legs towards the ceiling, maintaining control and avoiding swinging motions.
- Lower your legs back down without letting them swing.

Tips for Precise Execution:

1. Controlled Movements:
   - Focus on controlled and deliberate movements, ensuring that your lower abs are doing the work.

2. Maintain Core Engagement:
   - Throughout each exercise, keep your core engaged to maximize effectiveness and protect your lower back.

3. Breathing:
   - Coordinate your breath with the movements. Exhale during the effort phase and inhale during the relaxation phase.

4. Adjust Intensity:
   - Tailor the intensity based on your fitness level. Beginners may start with fewer repetitions or shorter durations, gradually progressing as strength increases.

As you embark on the realm of leg raises and lower ab workouts, visualize each repetition as a step towards a more defined and resilient lower core. Adjust the suggested durations based on your fitness level, and always prioritize proper form for effective results. Get ready to elevate your core strength and unveil the power of your lower abs!

Core-Strengthening Equipment:
Unleashing the Power Within

Welcome to a chapter that introduces game-changing equipment into your core-strengthening arsenal. In this chapter, we'll explore the transformative benefits of stability balls and resistance bands, providing you with tools that can elevate your core workouts for better and faster results. Discover how incorporating these pieces of equipment can revolutionize your approach to core enhancement, along with suggested durations and precise execution techniques.

1. Stability Balls: Dynamic Core Engagement

Stability balls, also known as Swiss balls, introduce an element of instability, making them excellent tools for challenging and enhancing your core workouts.

Benefits:

- Enhanced Core Activation: The unstable surface of the stability ball engages deeper core muscles, intensifying your workout.

- Improved Balance and Coordination: Performing exercises on the ball challenges your balance, promoting coordination and stability.

- Versatility in Exercises: From basic crunches to planks, stability balls offer a versatile platform for a range of core workouts.

Workout Duration:

- Beginner: 15-20 minutes

- Intermediate: 20-30 minutes

- Advanced: 30 minutes or more

Execution:

- Stability Ball Crunches:

- Sit on the ball with your feet flat on the floor.

- Perform crunches, lifting your upper body while keeping the ball stable.

- Plank with Feet on Ball:

- Start in a plank position with your feet on the stability ball.

- Hold the plank, engaging your core to maintain stability.

2. Resistance Bands: Targeted Resistance Amplified
Resistance bands are versatile tools that add controlled resistance to your exercises, focusing on specific muscle groups and enhancing your core strength.
Benefits:
  - Targeted Resistance: Resistance bands isolate and intensify the engagement of core muscles, fostering strength and endurance.
  - Portable and Versatile: Compact and easy to carry, resistance bands allow you to include core workouts anywhere, anytime.
  - Gradual Progression: Multiple resistance levels enable progressive challenges for continuous core development.
Workout Duration:
  - Beginner: 15-20 minutes
  - Intermediate: 20-30 minutes
  - Advanced: 30 minutes or more
Execution:
  - Standing Oblique Crunch with Band:
    - Attach the band to a fixed point.
    - Pull the band while crunching to the side, engaging your obliques.
  - Seated Russian Twists with Band:
    - Sit on the floor with legs extended.
    - Hold the band and perform Russian twists, engaging your entire core.
3. Bosu Balance Trainer: Core Stability Amplified
The Bosu Balance Trainer introduces dynamic stability training, challenging your core through its unique flat-dome design.

Benefits:

- Dynamic Stability Training: The Bosu's instability activates stabilizing muscles, providing a dynamic and effective core workout.

- Improved Proprioception: Enhances body awareness and coordination, crucial for overall balance.

- Diverse Exercise Options:Bosu offers a variety of exercises to engage the entire core.

Workout Duration:

Beginner: 15-20 minutes

Intermediate: 20-30 minutes

Advanced: 30 minutes or more

Execution:

Bosu Ball Plank:

- Place forearms on the flat side of the Bosu.

- Hold a plank position, engaging your core to stabilize.

Bosu Ball Squats:

- Stand on the flat side of the Bosu.

- Perform squats, engaging your core for stability.

Tips for Incorporating Equipment:

1. Start Gradually:

- Introduce equipment gradually, ensuring you are comfortable with the movements before progressing to more challenging exercises.

2. Focus on Form:

- Prioritize proper form to maximize the benefits of each exercise and reduce the risk of injury.

3. Adapt to Your Fitness Level:
   - Choose resistance levels and stability challenges that align with your current fitness level. As you progress, increase the intensity.

 Elevate Your Core Journey
With stability balls, resistance bands, and Bosu Balance Trainers at your disposal, your core-strengthening journey takes on a new dimension. Embrace the challenge, explore the versatility, and let the synergy between you and these tools sculpt a core that radiates strength and resilience. Your journey to a more robust core just reached new heights—enjoy the ascent!

Core-Friendly Nutrition:
Nourishing the Strength Within

Welcome to a chapter dedicated to understanding the pivotal role of nutrition in fortifying your core strength and promoting overall fitness. As you've embarked on this journey to sculpt a resilient core, it's crucial to recognize that what you fuel your body with plays a significant role in achieving your goals. Let's delve into the principles of core-friendly nutrition and outline a suggested nutrition plan that complements your efforts.

The Foundation: Understanding Core-Friendly Nutrition

1. Hydration Matters:

- Adequate water intake is foundational for overall health and crucial for maintaining the elasticity of muscles, including your core muscles.

2. Protein Power:

- Protein is the building block for muscle repair and growth. Include lean protein sources such as poultry, fish, tofu, and legumes in your diet.

3. Healthy Fats for Sustained Energy:

- Incorporate sources of healthy fats like avocados, nuts, and olive oil. These fats provide sustained energy for your workouts.

4. Complex Carbohydrates:

- Opt for complex carbohydrates such as whole grains, sweet potatoes, and quinoa to provide a steady release of energy during your training sessions.

5. Nutrient-Rich Foods:

- Ensure a diverse intake of fruits and vegetables to provide essential vitamins, minerals, and antioxidants that support overall health and recovery.

The Core Nutrition Plan: Fueling Your Strength

Morning Fuel (Pre-Workout):
   - Option 1: Greek yogurt with berries and a sprinkle of chia seeds.
   - Option 2: Oatmeal topped with sliced banana and a spoonful of almond butter.

Post-Workout Refuel:
   - Option 1: Protein smoothie with whey protein, spinach, banana, and almond milk.
   - Option 2: Grilled chicken or tofu wrap with whole-grain tortilla and plenty of veggies.

Midday Nourishment:
   - Option 1: Quinoa salad with mixed vegetables, chickpeas, and a light vinaigrette.
   - Option 2: Salmon or tempeh with sweet potato and steamed broccoli.

Afternoon Snack:
   - Option 1: Greek yogurt parfait with granola and mixed berries.
   - Option 2: Handful of almonds or walnuts with an apple.

Evening Sustenance:
   - Option 1: Grilled turkey or plant-based burger with a side of quinoa and roasted vegetables.

- Option 2: Stir-fried tofu or shrimp with brown rice and a variety of colorful stir-fried vegetables.

Before Bed (Optional):
  - Option 1: Cottage cheese with sliced peaches.
  - Option 2: Herbal tea with a small handful of mixed nuts.

Nutrition Tips for Core Enhancement:

1. Balanced Macros:
   - Ensure a balanced intake of carbohydrates, proteins, and fats to support energy levels and muscle recovery.

2. Timing Matters:
   - Consume a balance of macronutrients around your workouts, emphasizing protein for muscle repair.

3. Hydration Habit:
   - Maintain adequate hydration throughout the day. Water is essential for cellular function and overall health.

4. Mindful Eating:
   - Practice mindful eating to foster a healthy relationship with food. Pay attention to hunger and fullness cues.

5. Supplementation Support:
   - Consider consulting with a healthcare professional for personalized advice on supplements such as vitamins or omega-3 fatty acids.

Nourish, Strengthen, Thrive

As you embark on this journey of core enhancement, remember that nutrition is your ally in reaching your fitness goals. Embrace the power of whole, nutrient-dense foods to fuel your workouts, support muscle recovery, and fortify the strength within. This nutrition plan is a foundation for your core-friendly eating habits—customize it based on your preferences and dietary needs. Here's to nourishing your core and thriving in every step of your fitness journey!

Advanced Core Workouts: *Pushing Boundaries for Peak Strength*

Congratulations on reaching the pinnacle of your core-strengthening journey! In this chapter, we'll explore advanced and intense workouts designed to challenge your core muscles at the highest level. Whether you're an experienced fitness enthusiast or someone ready to take their core training to the next level, these exercises will push your boundaries and elevate your strength. Let's dive into advanced workouts, detailing their execution, suggested durations, and the specific core parts they target.

1. Dragon Flags: Sculpting Superwoman Abs

Execution:

- Lie on your back on a bench or flat surface, holding onto the bench behind your head.
- Lift your legs and lower back off the bench, keeping your body straight.
- Lower your legs back down without letting them touch the bench.

Duration: 5 sets of 20 reps

Targeted Core Part:
- Primarily targets the rectus abdominis.

2. Hanging Windshield Wipers: Advanced Oblique Challenge

Execution:
- Hang from a pull-up bar with your arms fully extended.
- Lift your legs to one side, bringing them towards your hands.
- Lower your legs to the other side without letting them touch the ground.

Duration: 5 sets of 20 reps (each side)

Targeted Core Part:
- Intensely engages the obliques.

3. V-Ups: Total Core Activation

Execution:
- Lie on your back with arms extended overhead.

- Simultaneously lift your legs and upper body, forming a V shape.
    - Lower your legs and upper body back down without letting them touch the ground.

Duration: 5 sets of 25 reps

Targeted Core Part:
    - Engages the entire core, with emphasis on the rectus abdominis.

4. Plank with Alternating Leg and Arm Lifts: Dynamic Stability Challenge

Execution:
    - Start in a plank position.
    - Lift one leg and the opposite arm simultaneously while maintaining a straight body.
    - Lower them back down and repeat on the other side.

Duration: 5 sets of 20 reps (each side)

Targeted Core Part:
    - Challenges overall core stability, with focus on the lower back and glutes.

5. Medicine Ball Russian Twists with Leg Raise: Coordination and Strength Fusion

Execution:
    - Sit on the floor holding a medicine ball.

- Perform a Russian twist, bringing the ball to each side.
- As you twist to one side, lift your legs off the ground.

Duration: 5 sets of 25 reps (each side)

Targeted Core Part:
- Engages the obliques, rectus abdominis, and hip flexors.

Tips for Advanced Core Workouts:

1. Progress Gradually:
- Gradually increase the intensity and volume of these exercises to avoid overtraining.

2. Maintain Form:
- Prioritize form over quantity. Perform each repetition with controlled and deliberate movements.

3. Listen to Your Body:
- Pay attention to your body's signals. If an exercise causes pain beyond the normal discomfort of a challenging workout, reassess your form or consider modifications.

4. Include Recovery Days:
- Ensure sufficient rest and recovery days between intense core workouts to allow your muscles to repair and grow stronger.

As you incorporate these advanced core workouts into your routine, remember that mastery comes with time and consistency. Push your limits, celebrate your progress, and revel in the strength you're cultivating within your core. This chapter marks a new chapter in your fitness journey—embrace the challenge and revel in the transformation!

Consistency and Progress Tracking: *Your Path to Lasting Transformation*

In the realm of core enhancement, consistency is the cornerstone upon which lasting transformation is built. This chapter explores the profound significance of maintaining a consistent workout routine and introduces practical tools for tracking your progress. Let's delve into the importance of consistency and unveil a day-by-day tracking table to empower you on your journey to a stronger and more resilient core.

The Power of Consistency

1. Building Habits:

- Consistency transforms actions into habits. Regular engagement with your core workouts ingrains them into your daily routine.

2. Incremental Progress:
   - Small, consistent efforts accumulate over time, leading to significant progress. Consistency is the key to unlocking your full potential.

3. Muscle Adaptation:
   - Consistent training allows your muscles to adapt and strengthen. The more regularly you challenge your core, the more resilient and powerful it becomes.

4. Mental Resilience:
   - Consistency nurtures mental resilience. Overcoming daily challenges builds mental fortitude, empowering you to push through barriers.

The Tracking Table: Your Visual Progress Journal

Embark on a transformative journey by incorporating a day-by-day tracking table into your routine. This simple yet powerful tool provides a visual representation of your consistency and progress.

Day	Workout Type	Duration	Intensity	Feelings/Notes
1	[Exercise Name]	[XX minutes]	[Low/Medium/High]	[How you felt]

2	[Exercise Name]	[XX minutes]	[Low/Medium/High]	[How you felt]
3	[Exercise Name]	[XX minutes]	[Low/Medium/High]	[How you felt]
...	...	...	...	...

How to Use the Tracking Table:

1. Exercise Name:
   - Specify the core exercises you performed on each day.

2. Duration:
   - Record the time spent on your core workouts.

3. Intensity:
   - Rate the intensity of your workout on a scale of Low/Medium/High.

4. Feelings/Notes:
   - Reflect on how you felt during and after each workout. Include any notes or observations.

Tips for Utilizing the Tracking Table:

1. Daily Consistency:

- Aim to fill out the tracking table every day, fostering a sense of daily accountability.

2. Honest Self-Reflection:
   - Be honest in rating the intensity and capturing your feelings. This aids in adjusting your workouts based on your energy levels and progress.

3. Celebrate Milestones:
   - Periodically review your tracking table to celebrate milestones and identify patterns in your progress.

4. Adapt and Evolve:
   - Use the information gathered to adapt your routine. If a particular exercise consistently leaves you energized, consider incorporating it more frequently.

Conclusion: Your Journey Unfolds Day by Day

Consistency, coupled with diligent progress tracking, propels you towards your core-strengthening goals. The day-by-day tracking table is not just a record; it's a visual testament to your commitment and growth. As you fill in each cell, remember that every tick is a step towards a more powerful, resilient core. Embrace the journey, celebrate your consistency, and watch as the days add up to a transformative story of strength and endurance. This chapter marks a pivotal point—your path to lasting transformation awaits.

Embracing Triumph: A Celebration of Your Core Journey

As we conclude this empowering guide to core enhancement, it's time to reflect on the key points, renew your commitment, and celebrate the remarkable achievements along your path to a stronger and more resilient core.

Summarizing the Journey

1. Consistency is Key:
   - Consistent engagement with your core workouts transforms efforts into habits, paving the way for lasting transformation.

2. Holistic Approach to Nutrition:
   - Nourish your body with a balanced diet, emphasizing protein, healthy fats, and nutrient-rich foods to support overall health and core strength.

3. Progressive Workouts:
   - Gradually progress from foundational exercises to advanced workouts, challenging your core muscles to adapt and grow stronger.

4. Diverse Exercises and Equipment:
   - Integrate a variety of exercises and core-strengthening equipment to keep your routine dynamic, engaging different muscle groups for comprehensive development.

5. Mindful Tracking and Reflection:

- Utilize the day-by-day tracking table as a tool for self-reflection, celebrating successes, and adjusting your routine based on progress and feelings.

A Call to Commitment

As you stand at this juncture, fueled by the knowledge and dedication you've invested, recommit to your core journey. Embrace each workout as an opportunity to sculpt not just your physical strength but also your mental resilience. Understand that setbacks are part of the journey, and every challenge you overcome is a victory in itself.

Celebrating Your Triumphs

1. Acknowledge Every Tick:
   - Celebrate each tick on your tracking table as a testament to your consistency and determination.

2. Milestones Matter:
   - Recognize and celebrate milestones, whether it's an increased workout duration, mastering a challenging exercise, or simply maintaining a consistent routine.

3. Reflect on Transformations:
   - Take a moment to reflect on the transformations—both physical and mental—that have unfolded throughout your core-strengthening journey.

Your Core Journey is an Ongoing Triumph

This guide is not just a collection of exercises and tips; it's a roadmap to triumph—one that is ongoing and ever-evolving. Your core journey is a celebration of your commitment, resilience, and the continuous pursuit of becoming the strongest version of yourself.

Your Core Triumph Awaits

As you close this chapter and continue your journey, remember that triumph is not solely found in the destination but in every step taken, every challenge faced, and every victory achieved along the way. Your core, now a symbol of strength and resilience, awaits further triumphs. Embrace the journey, stay committed, and revel in the triumph that is uniquely yours. The final chapter marks the beginning of a new phase—your core triumph awaits!